The Under The Tree Serie

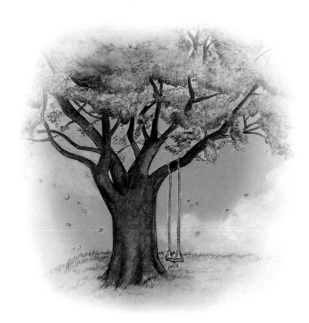

Waiting For Emma: A Brother's Story
(For Siblings and Families with Babies in the NICU)

Written By Danielle Leibovici, LMFT
Illustrated By Julia Gabrielov

Dedicated to babies everywhere who have spent time in the NICU or hospital in their first year of life. You are fighting warriors who touch our lives ever so deepl

Dedicated to families everywhere who have spent time in the NICU or hospital during their baby's first year of life. I honor your bravery, vulnerability, and endurance

Published by Bloom Publishing, 417 West 20st. #11451 Norfolk, Virginia
The Under The Tree Series ™
Text Copyright © 2014 by Danielle Leibovici
Illustration Copyright © 2014 by Danielle Leibovici
Distributed through Bloom Publishing

0-9857939-3-7

ISBN-:978-0-9857939-3-7

Library of Congress Number: 2014947813

Requests for permission to make copies of any part of the work should be sent through the below website: DanielleLeibovici.com

For information about custom editions, fundraising campaigns, speaking engagements, and author's visits, please send an email to info@danielleleibovici.com

Dear NICU Family and Friends,

After giving birth at the hospital, I never expected to be driving with an empty car seat while following an ambulance to the closest NICU for my newborn to get lifesaving treatment. Despite her being a full-term baby with an easy delivery, this is what happened when our second daughter, Aura, was born. Right away, our world shrank, and our measurement of time was centered around updated lab tests every four hours. Just hours earlier I was holding her close in my arms. Now, I found myself in the NICU, my baby in an incubator with wires everywhere. All I could do was stroke her cheek and sing to her. I slept in the pump-room adjacent to the NICU for four days just to be near Aura. I continued to pump breast milk for when she would be able to nurse. Fortunately, five days later, Aura was discharged with a clean bill of health.

Although we were at the NICU a relatively short amount of time, that experience profoundly changed our lives. I was able to get to know the doctors and nurses on a personal and very vulnerable level. When they found out I was a family therapist and the author of the **Under the Tree** children's book series, they asked for my help in fulfilling a need. They asked me to write a book to benefit siblings and families who were not prepared for the NICU. I took their request seriously and personally. As a result, *Waiting for Emma: A Brother's Story (For Siblings and Families with Babies in the NICU)* was created for families just like yours.

With this story, I wanted to remind all readers about the virtues of waiting. When I was in the NICU, I couldn't yet grasp that this painful experience would someday be far behind our family. *Waiting for Emma* is filled with resources, gentle support, and hope. Today, Aura is one of the happiest and most delightful of children. May this book bring a sense of connection and understanding, and a new perception of time for you and your family. When you are better supported, your baby will be, too.

May love and healing be with you.

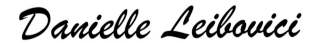

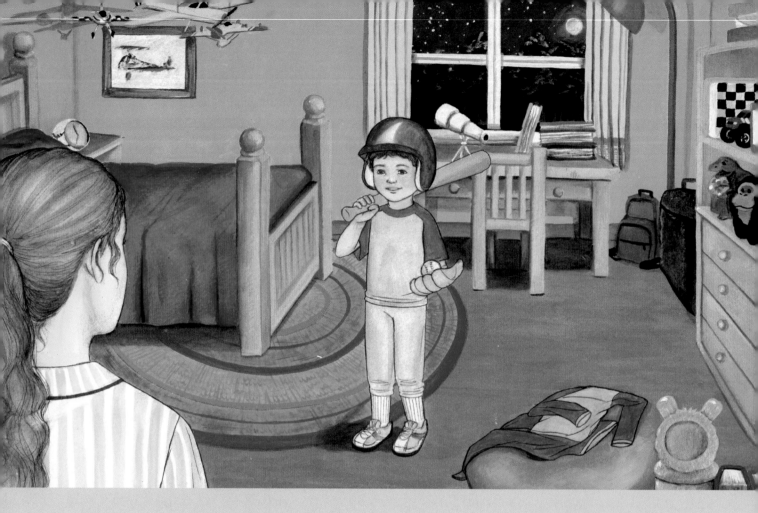

"Mom, I am ready to play baseball now!" Adam announced.

His mother looked at him and smiled. He was dressed from head to toe in his baseball uniform. Adam had his helmet on, his glove in one hand and the bat in the other. There was only one small problem.

It was nighttime.

"Honey, I see that you are all ready to go, but we can't play now silly. It's dark outside!"

"So I'll play in the dark," he replied.

"Well, how will you see where the bases are? And who would you play with at this time of night?"

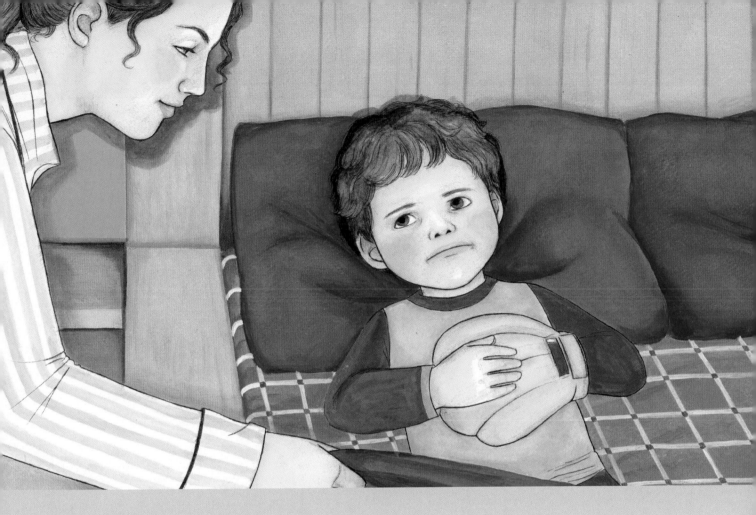

Adam's shoulders slumped. He hadn't thought about that. He didn't want to wait until morning. He just wanted to have fun and play baseball now.

His mother walked him to his bed. "It's good that we have the nighttime sweetheart, that's when we get our rest. Without bedtime, we wouldn't have energy for the next day. You need lots of energy to play baseball, right?"

"I guess so," Adam said, but he was still not happy about it. He took off his helmet.

His mother kissed him goodnight and Adam went to sleep.

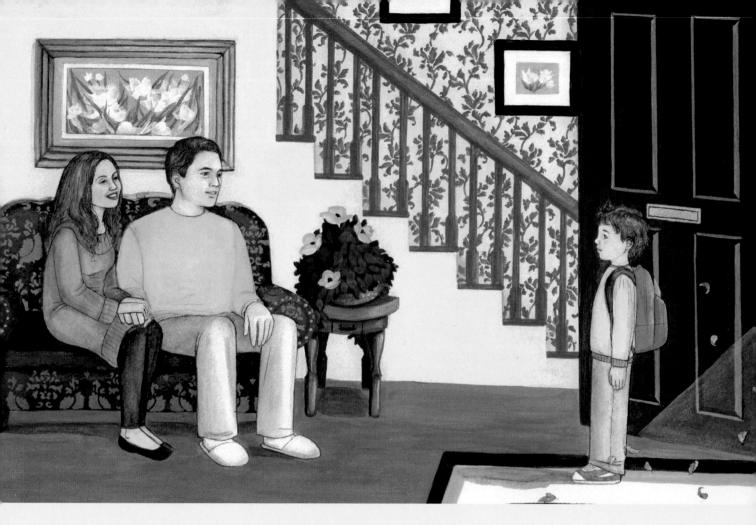

One special afternoon, Adam came home from school to find his parents sitting on the couch waiting for him.

"Honey, come here. Mommy and Daddy have something to tell you."

"What is it?" he asked.

"Remember when you asked me when you would ever get to be a big brother?" His mother smiled.

"Yes," he replied.

"Well, guess what? You are going to get your wish! You are going to be a big brother to a little baby sister or baby brother!"

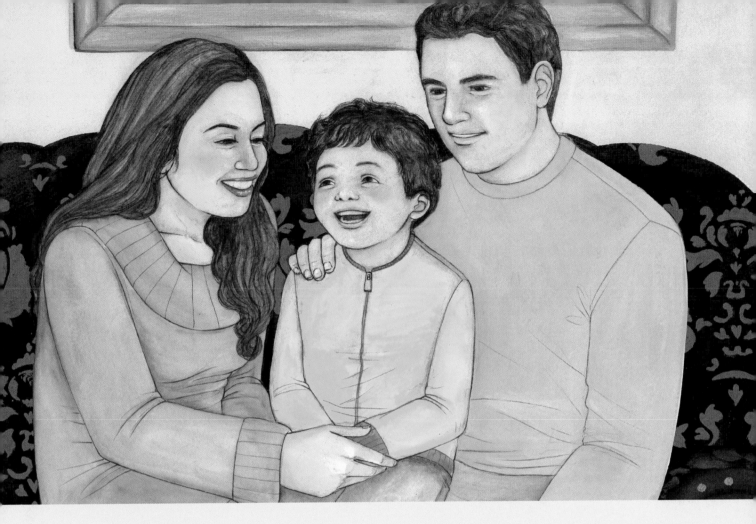

"Great!" Adam shouted. "Where is the baby?" He got up to search.

His parents laughed.

"The baby isn't here yet, but he or she is growing safely in a special place in Mommy's belly, and in June when school is out, the baby will be here."

"Ahhh, I have to wait that long!"

"Well," said his mother, "It's good to wait these months, since that gives the baby time to grow and be ready to be born. Besides, don't you want to see how funny Mommy is going to look with a big belly?"

Adam smiled, "I guess that is going to be funny!"

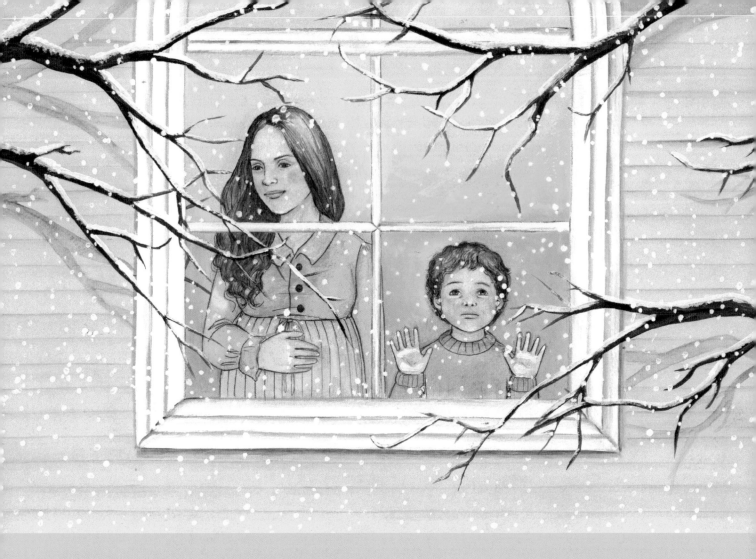

Mommy's belly was definitely getting bigger.

"Mom, it's cold outside. Why does it have to snow so much? I can't play baseball in the snow," Adam sighed.

She looked out the window with him.

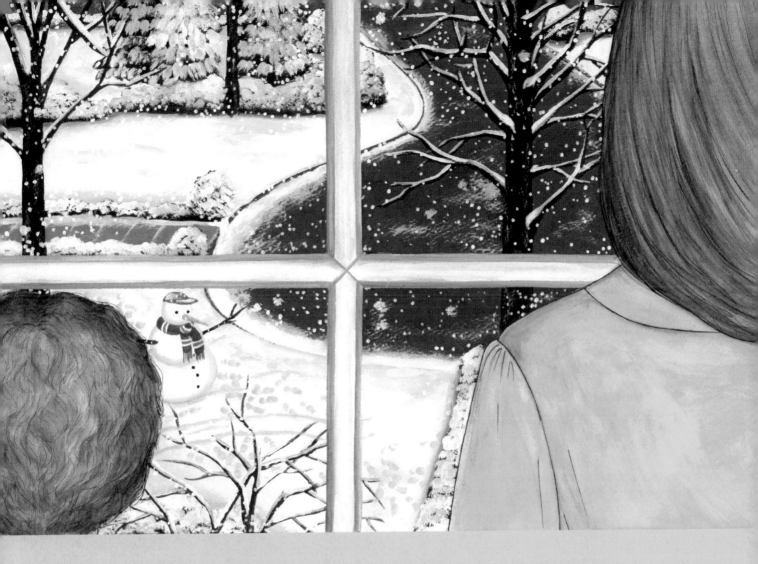

"Well, we need the winter to help the trees get ready for spring. And spring is when you play baseball, right?"

"Yeah, but why do I have to wait so long," he whined.

"It's good that we have the winter, because the cold helps the old leaves fall off the trees so new ones can come in. And wasn't that you the other day, having a big snowball fight with Daddy?"

He smiled. Yes, it was. He sure got Dad good!

Adam felt better. He went to play in his room.

Spring was finally here!

Adam came home from playing baseball. He was surprised to see his grandma waiting for him. He was very happy to see her!

"Hi, Grandma! What are you doing here?" he asked, giving her a hug.

"Hi, honey! It looks like your baby sister wanted to come a little early," she said.

"A baby sister! Where is she?" he exclaimed.

"Well, the baby will have to stay a little bit longer at the hospital in a place called the NICU, which is a word that sounds like nick-you."

"The NICU?" Adam repeated as he scratched his head. He wondered what that was.

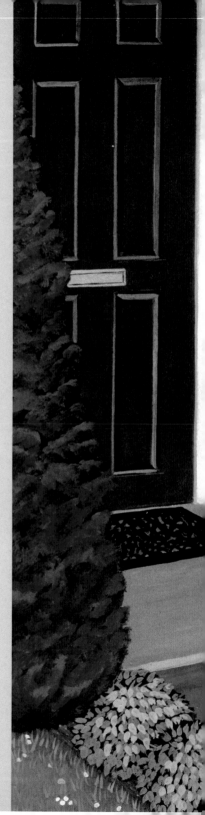

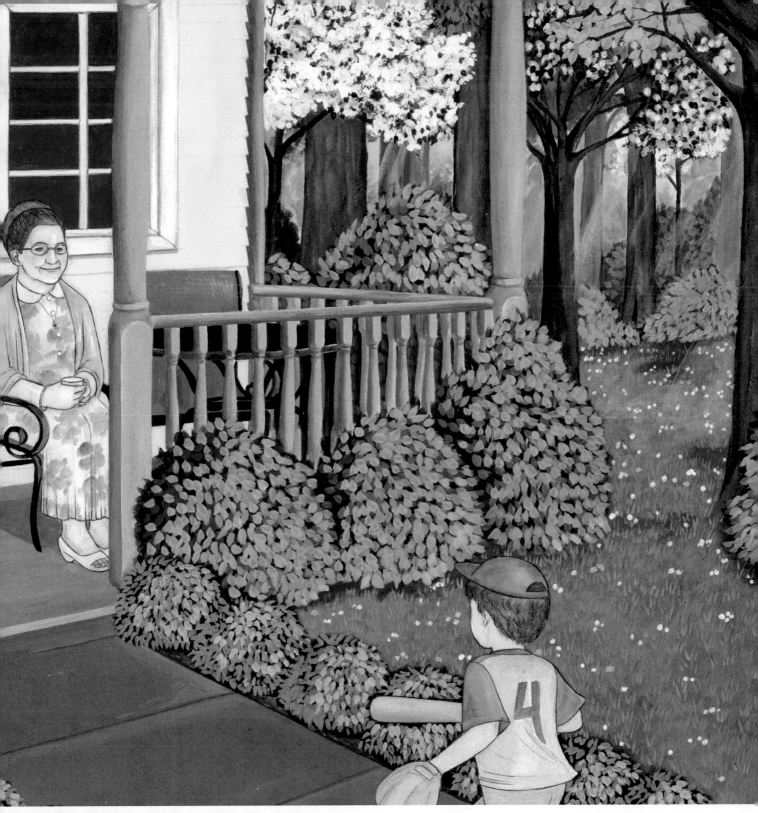

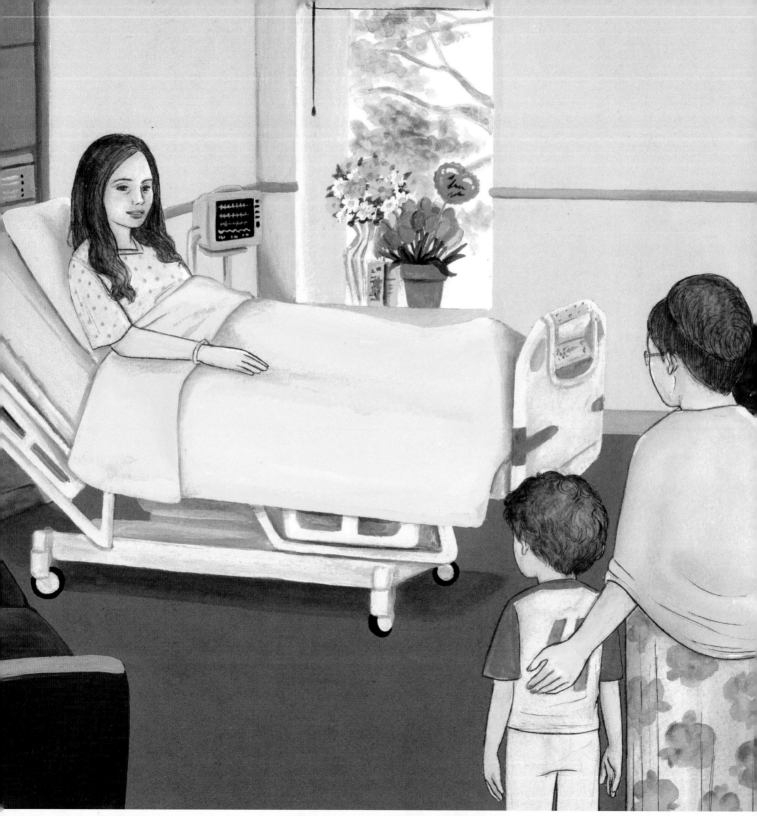

In the hospital, Adam's mom was sitting up in her bed.

"Hi, Mommy, where is my baby sister?"

"Hi, sweetheart! Yes, your baby sister is out of mommy's belly. Her name is Emma. We named her that because it means 'faith.' She is in the NICU, and Daddy is there with her."

"What is the NICU?" Adam asked.

"NICU stands for Neonatal Intensive Care Unit, and it is a special place where very smart doctors and nurses will take care of her until she is big enough and strong enough to come home. Emma wanted to come out a little earlier than we thought. I guess she was in a rush to meet us!"

"But why can't she get bigger and stronger at our home?" Adam wanted to know.

His mother took him in her arms. "The truth is that Mommy and Daddy don't like waiting either. We also wish your baby sister could come home now, but sometimes waiting is not such a terrible thing."

Remember that night you got all dressed up to play baseball and you didn't want to wait until morning to play? Then you agreed to wait and get a good night's sleep. That next day, you had the best game ever and hit two home runs!"

Adam smiled. He remembered.

"And remember when it was still winter outside, you wanted it to be spring so you could start playing baseball again? Then you decided to make the most of the wonderful snow, and it was spring before you knew it."

He smiled again. "That's true."

"I know we all want your sister home with us now. But it's good that we have the NICU, because it is a place just for very small babies to grow. They will help Emma get stronger more quickly. We do have to wait. But, in the meantime, we can visit her there as much as we like. You can even bring her a special toy or stuffed animal she can have near her while she gets bigger."

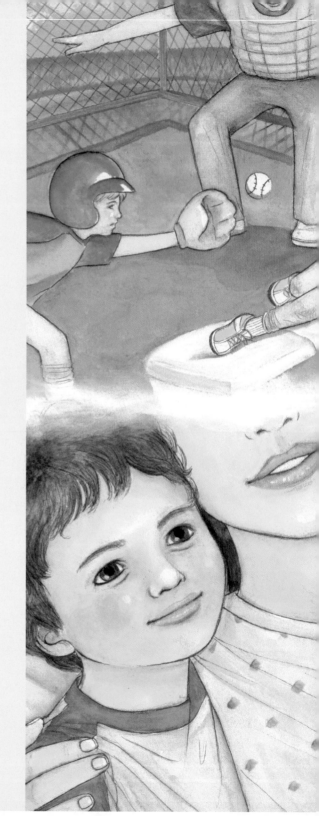

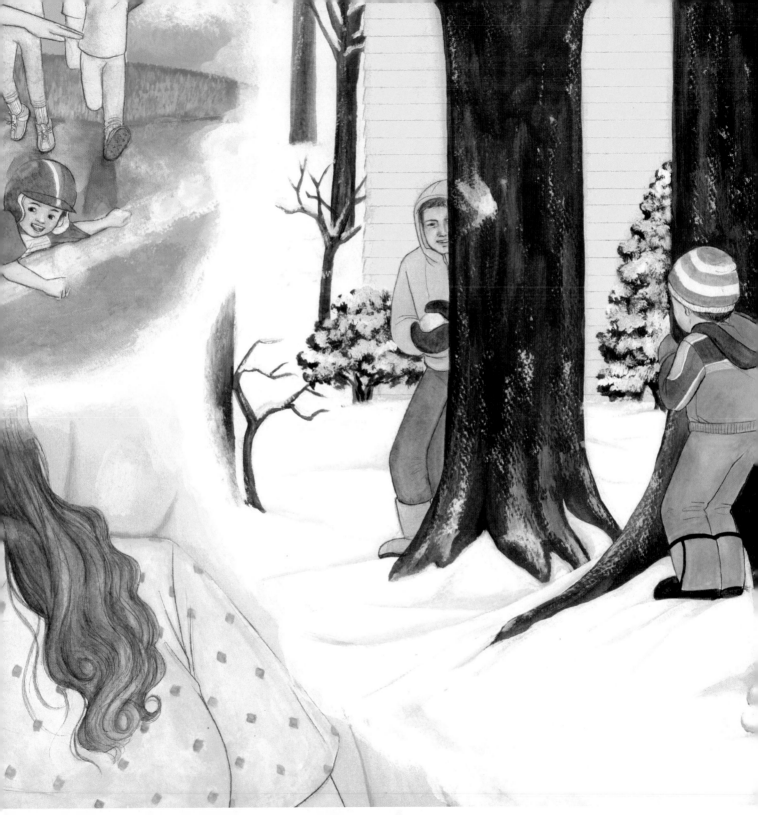

Adam thought about it. "Well, can I go and see her?"

"In a few more days, when your sister is comfortable, Daddy will take you to the NICU. In the meantime, I have a great idea. Can you draw a picture to hang close to where Emma will be sleeping?"

Adam thought about drawing his new sister a picture.

"I got it!" He knew exactly what he wanted to draw.

"Great, then get to it! Thank you for visiting me honey. I will see you soon."

Adam waved goodbye and went home with his dad and grandma.

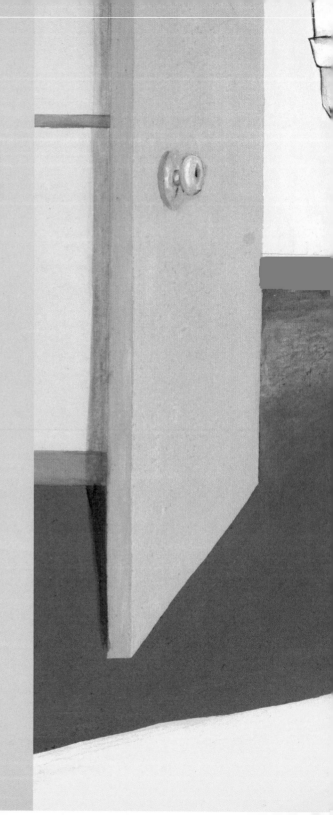

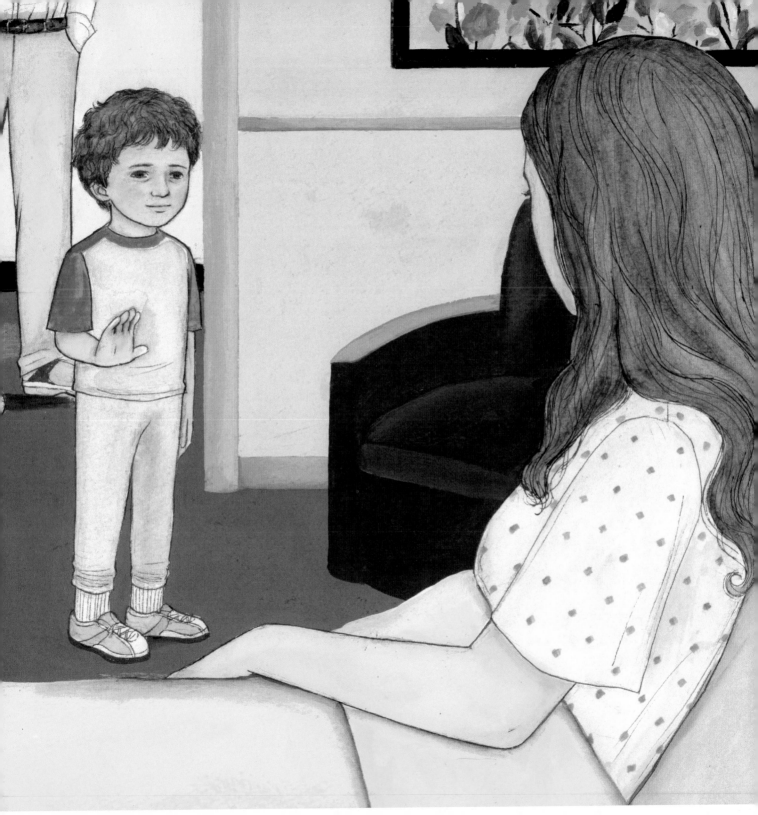

Two days later, Adam and his dad returned to the hospital.

"I want to tell you a little bit about this special room where Emma is staying," his dad said. "The NICU is a big room with lots of machines, lights, and noises. There are other babies in the room, too. When you get there, you will see some tubes and wires on your baby sister. Don't be scared. These tubes and wires are there to help her breathe and get stronger. They do not hurt her and they will be off as soon as she is ready."

Adam did not know what to expect.

Before they were able to go inside the NICU, Adam and his dad were told to wash their hands, pushing up their sleeves to wash all the way up to their elbows. His daddy even had to take off his watch.

A nurse helping them explained, "There are tiny things called germs that we don't want near brand-new babies."

Adam washed his hands. He thought it was funny that the sink had a pedal he could push with his feet to turn the water on.

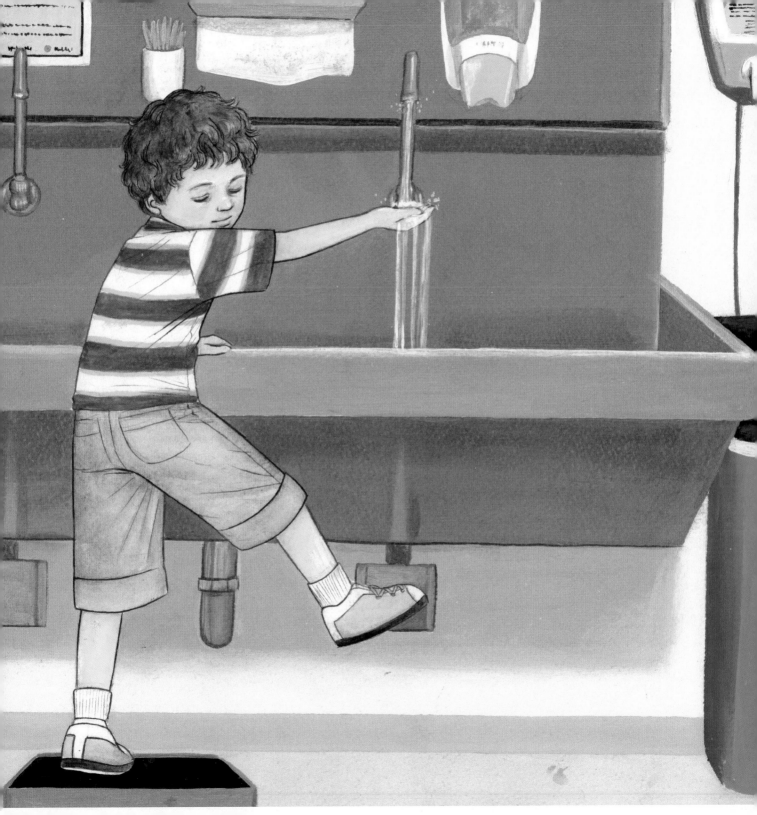

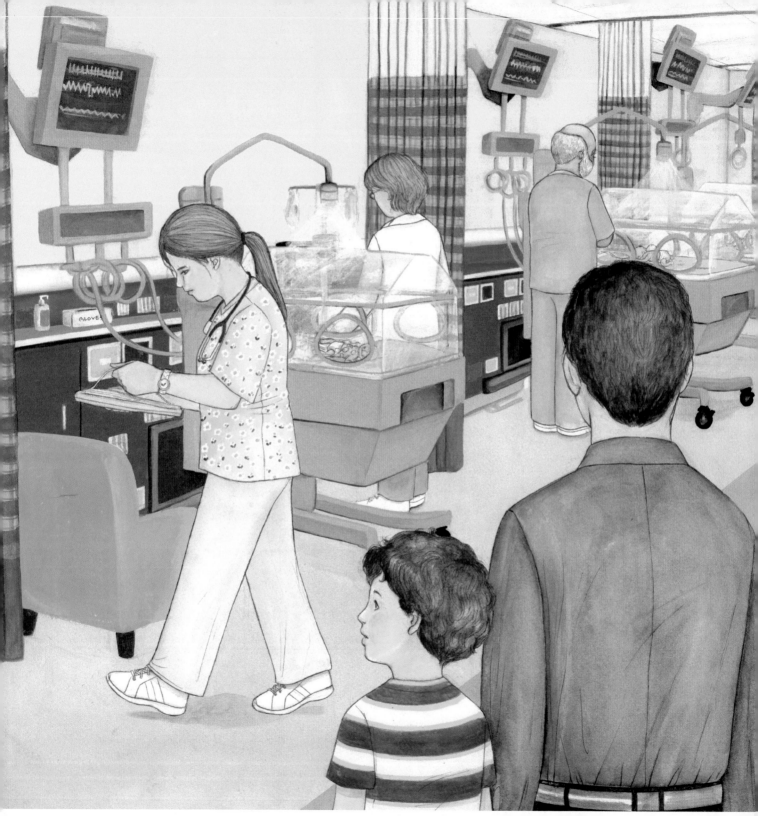

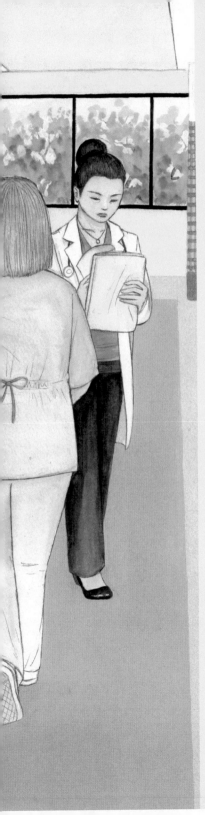

They stood in front of the doors of the NICU. The doors opened by themselves and Adam was now inside. The room was very noisy. He heard alarm bells going off and he saw big, loud machines. There were lights blinking on small screens everywhere. It was a little scary. He wanted to cover his ears. There were just so many machines with different-colored lights all over them. He looked around and saw little clear boxes, and could tell that babies must be in them. He saw wires that connected to the baby boxes. Some baby boxes had big machines and some did not. He wondered which baby was his sister.

Adam's daddy pointed in the direction of a baby's box.

"Is that Emma's box?" he asked his dad.

"Yes that is where she is sleeping right now. It does look like a box, but it is actually called an incubator and it keeps her nice and cozy. After all, she was in Mommy's belly for so long she still needs a snug, warm place to help her grow."

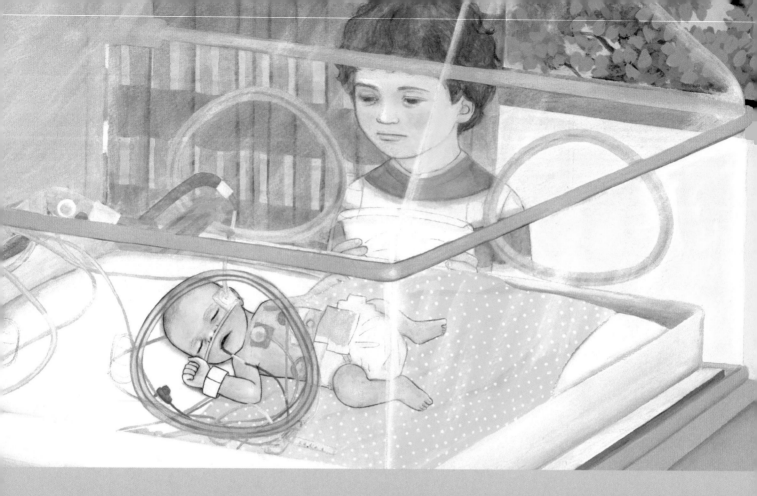

Adam saw Emma for the first time. She had wires on her chest and one wrist was connected to a brightly-buttoned machine. She looked very small to him and very wrinkly. Her eyes were shut tightly as she slept.

It bothered Adam that his baby sister had tubes and wires on her. Emma didn't look like his friend's baby sister, or the other babies he saw on TV. He wanted the tubes and wires off her now! He felt himself getting upset.

"Why did this happen to her Daddy? Why doesn't she look like a normal baby?" Adam asked.

"That is a good question, buddy. We sometimes don't know why these things happen," his daddy paused. "But, what we do know is that we love your baby sister, and we are glad she is here. The doctors and nurses are going to take good care of her until she gets big enough to come home. These next few

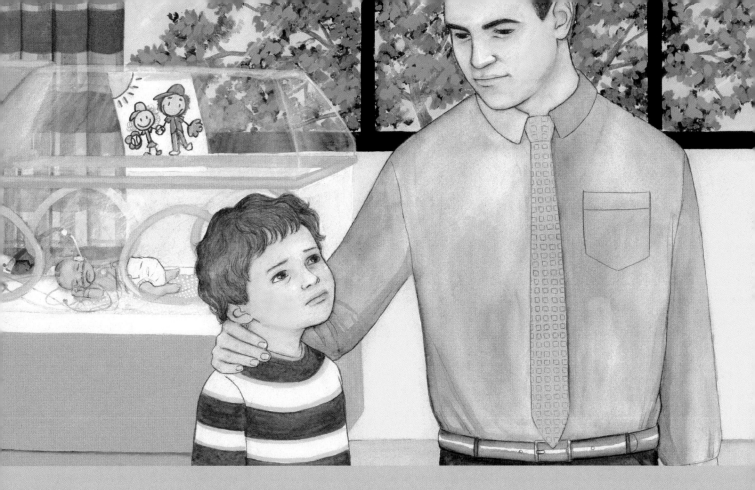

weeks will seem very long and may even be tough, but we will get through it because we are a strong family."

Adam had more questions, but he was ready to leave the NICU. He looked down at his baby sister.

"I love you Emma. Please hurry up and get better. I want to teach you how to play baseball."

Adam looked around the room. There were a lot of doctors and nurses with other little babies. Some of the doctors and nurses smiled at him. At least she won't be alone, he thought. He hung his picture next to Emma's incubator. Adam blew her a kiss and said goodbye, for now.

He went back home with one of her blankets.

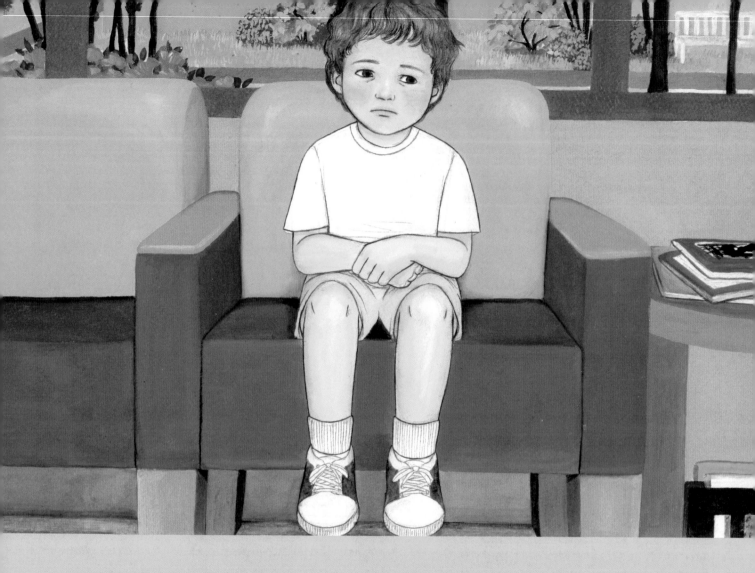

Waiting for Emma to get stronger was hard for Adam. It was hard for him to watch his parents spend all their free time at the hospital. They didn't have time for him like they used to. Many times Adam had to go to the hospital too. He hated that he had to be quiet while his parents talked to the doctors and nurses. It was hard for him to be there and stand still. He wanted to walk around. He wanted to touch Emma's arm, but he wasn't allowed to yet. All he could do was watch her sleep.

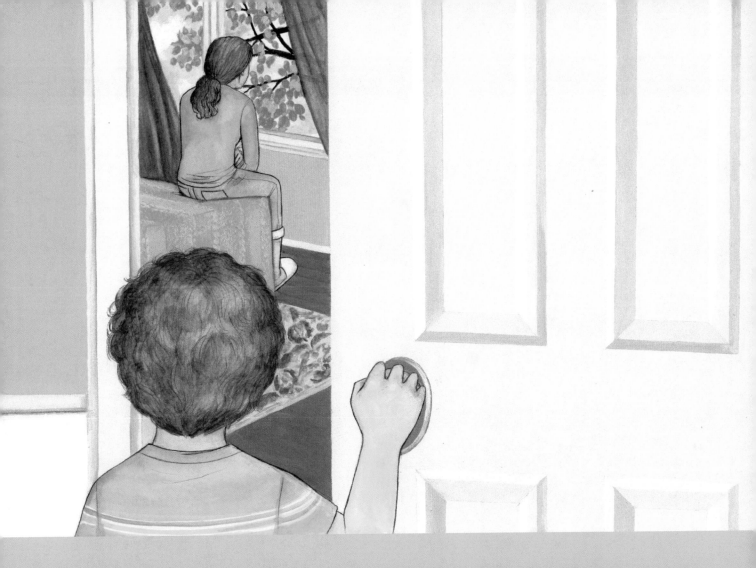

Some days, Adam would peek in on his mom when her door was closed. He saw that she looked sad. Adam didn't like to see his mom so sad. Sometimes when his dad would come home from work, he would talk to his mom and not play with Adam. Adam didn't like it when his dad didn't play with him.

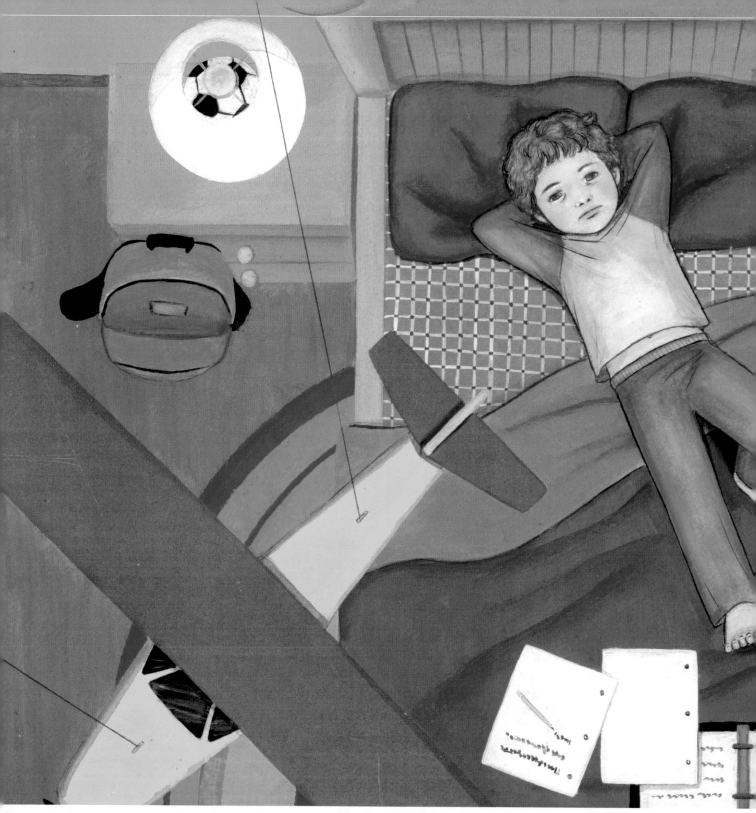

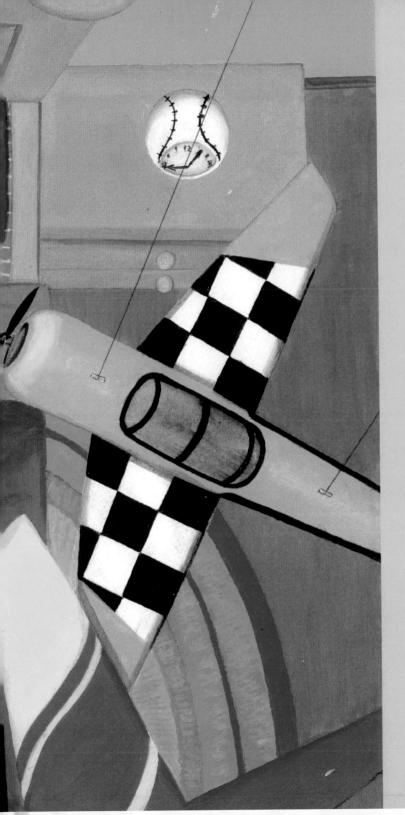

He wondered if his mom and dad cared as much for him as they did for the baby. Sometimes, he was even mad at his sister. Things were so different before Emma was born.

There were days when Adam would yell and scream and slam the door. He wished his life could be like it was before.

Weeks and weeks had passed. Why was it taking so long for Emma to get better?

The doctor xplained that baby Emma needed to reach these milestones before she could come home:

"First, we must wait until she can breathe on her own."

"Next, we must wait until her vital signs are stabilized."

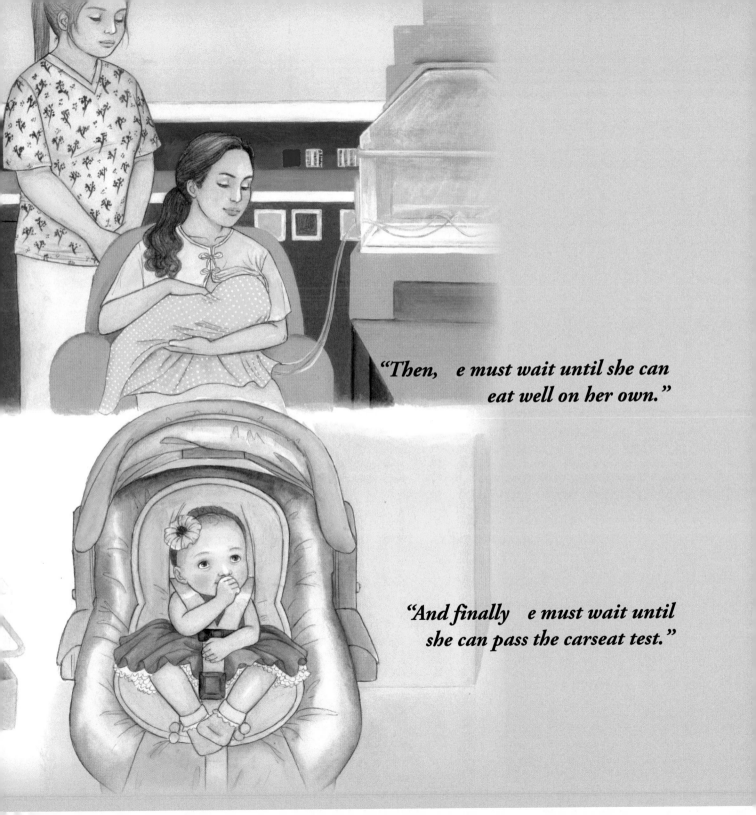

"Then, e must wait until she can eat well on her own."

"And finally e must wait until she can pass the carseat test."

Then one day, she was ready to leave the NICU.
Emma was coming home!

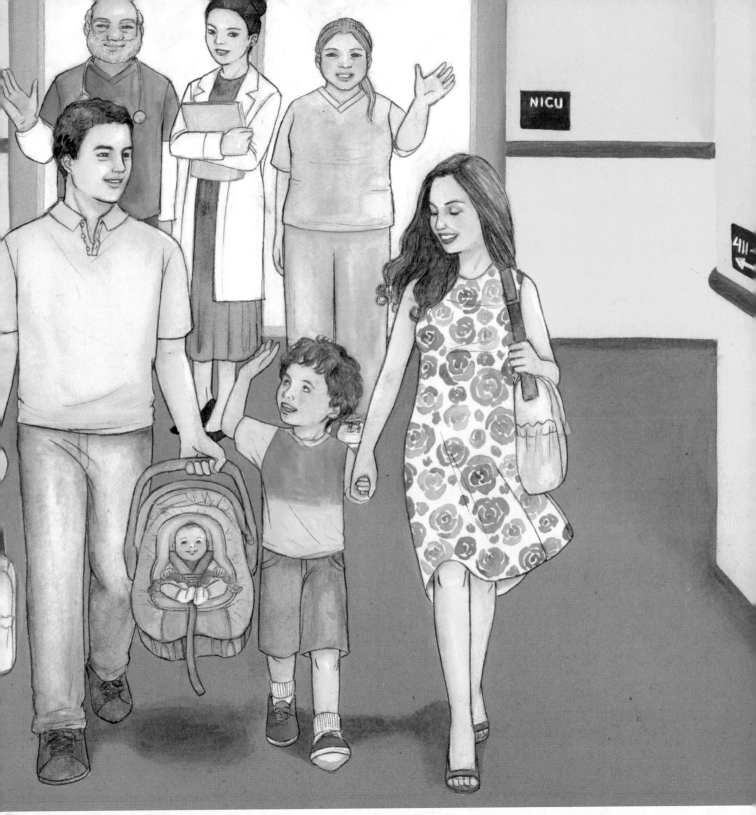

Adam had waited so long for Emma to come home. Now he had to wait even longer for her to get big enough to play baseball!

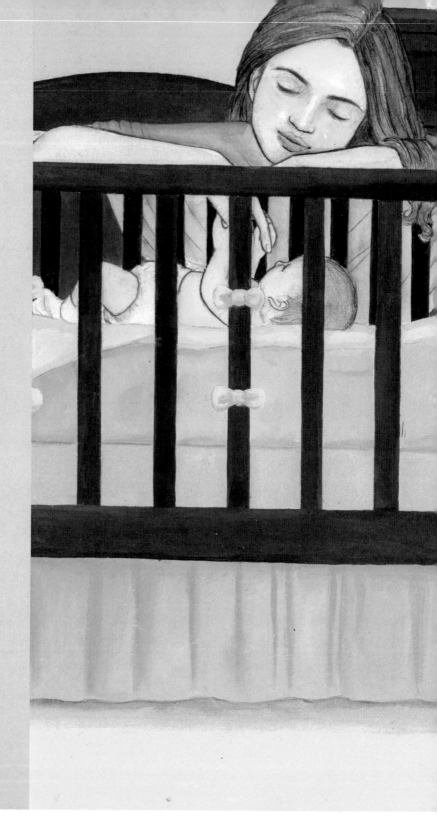

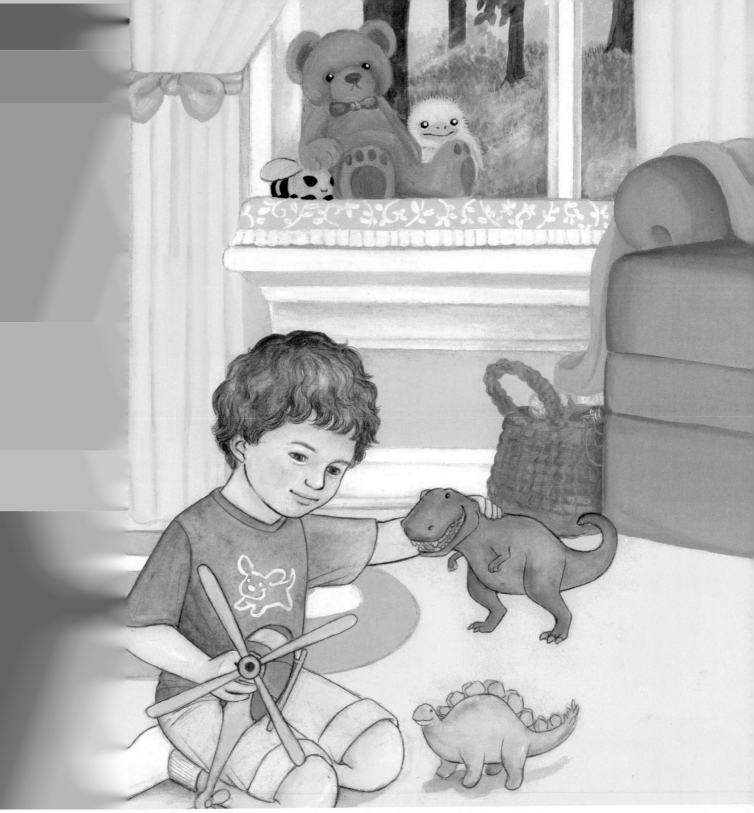

Emma got big enough! Adam taught her all that she needed to know about his favorite sport. He taught her how to catch, how to hit, and how to slide into the bases.

Emma loved baseball just as much as her big brother.

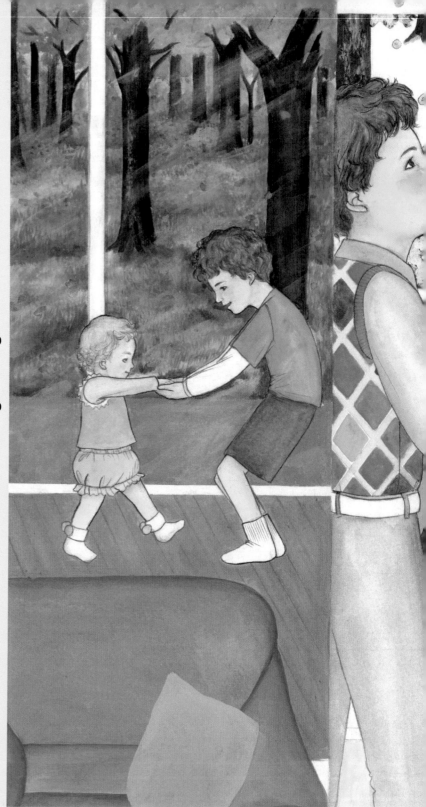

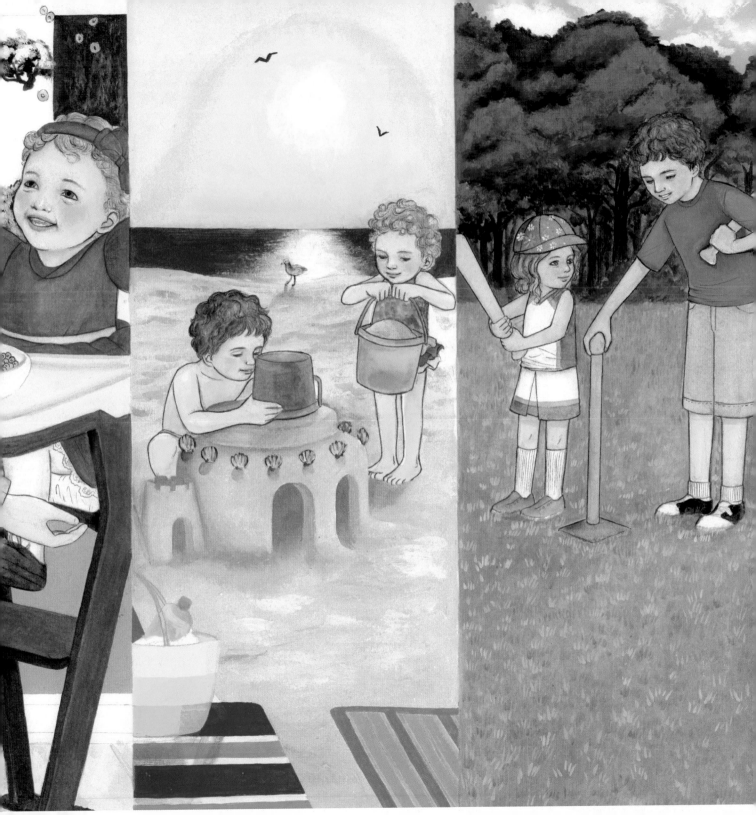

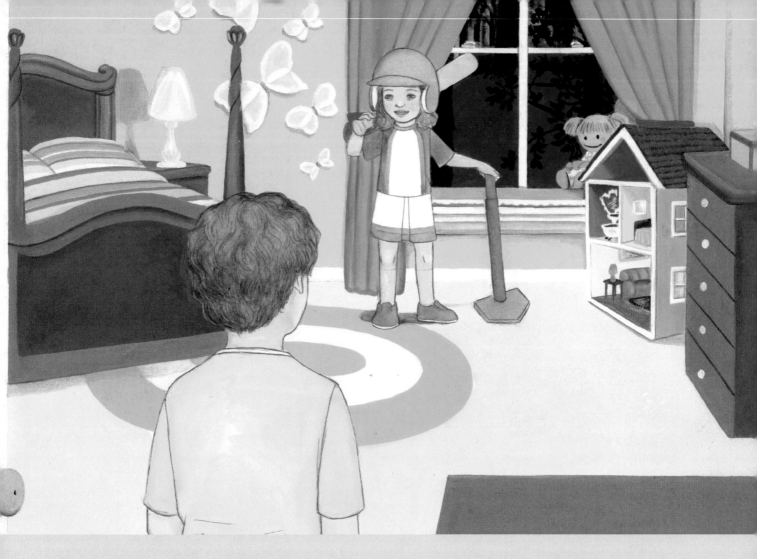

One night, Adam walked into his sister's room to say goodnight.

He burst out laughing. There Emma was, dressed from head to toe in her baseball uniform. She had her helmet on, held her glove in one hand, and the bat in the other. But it was time for bed.

"You are just like me," Adam smiled, "Even though it's dark outside, you can't wait to play baseball right? And I know you hate waiting!"

Emma nodded.

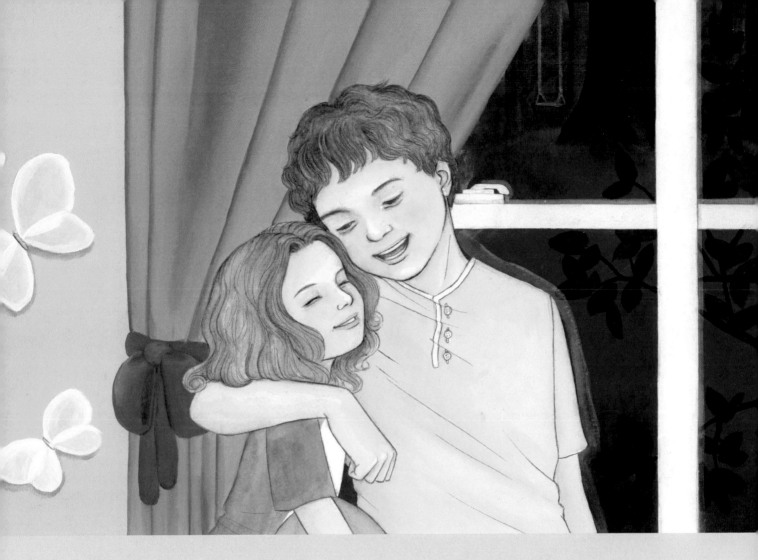

Adam looked down at his sister. She was so strong and healthy now and about to turn 5!

He put his arm around Emma's shoulders. "But sometimes sis, waiting brings you the best things."

The End

Understanding the Virtues of Waiting

When your child is in the NICU, nothing else seems as important. Your world may become very small as all your extra time and energy is now focused on the health and well-being of your preemie or newborn.

While I was in the NICU, I remember the nurses telling me not to be stressed as "the baby can sense a mother's duress." I thought to myself how absurd that was to hear! How could I not be stressed when my child was in this condition and all I could do was watch and pray for her to improve? A normal human reaction to something scary is to look for someone or something to blame. In order to gain more control over a stressful situation, we likely look for fault. Of course, many times we do not know why things happen the way they do (although we may spend much of our precious energy trying to make sense of it). Now is the time to put your energy into what you do know. You and your family know you are getting your baby the best care possible. You can be grateful for the NICU, with all the wonderful people there working around the clock to get your baby home. Your family also knows that you have even more strength and love to give when you come together and support each other in this process.

For Siblings:

With a baby in the NICU, it can be very easy to forget about the needs of your other child(ren). But remember, this unplanned circumstance is unexpected for your other child(ren) as well.

Siblings may misbehave more often because they are not getting the attention they were accustomed to before their younger sibling's birth. Children need individual attention and validation so they can learn to express themselves in positive ways. Also, a feeling of helplessness may exist for siblings, so making them part of the baby's action plan is a way to increase their con idence and security.

For Sharing:

By engaging in conversation, you let your child(ren) know their opinion matters, their experience matters, and most importantly, that they matter.

1. Do you have any questions about what is happening with your baby brother or sister? (And there is no such thing as a silly question.)

2. Mommy (or Daddy) feels (scared, mad, sad...) that your sister or brother is in the NICU. How do you feel?

3. Let's draw some pictures of how we are feeling about your baby brother or sister in the NICU. We can draw anything we want. Who is in the picture? Where are they? What are they doing? What are they feeling?

4. You can help your baby brother or sister, too! What do you think they would like to have next to them in bed to help them think of us? What kind of stuffed animal or blanket do you think they would like?

6. How can we make the time we visit your sister or brother better or easier for you? (Ideas may include age-appropriate incentives for when they sit quietly and allow you to speak to the doctors.)

7. What special activity can you and I do, just the two of us this weekend?

8. I understand that this may be hard for you to go through. I love you very much and am so proud of you for being baby _____'s big brother/sister. You are showing the baby how to be brave, patient, and loving. (Use any adjectives that would be suitable to affirm good behaviors and intentions.)

On Breastfeeding:

While in the NICU, you may feel helpless when it comes to the care of your own baby. You may only be able to watch as doctors and nurses meet their most basic needs, such as changing diapers or giving a bath. Breastfeeding, however, is a crucial contribution to a newborn's health and recovery which only a mother can give.

Breast milk supplies antibodies and cell-building properties vital to a more speedy recovery in the early stages of a preemie's life. Although formula does have calories, fat, and other added vitamins and nutrients, it cannot replace the individually specific benefits of breast milk for your newborn. Surprisingly, many preemies are often ready to practice nursing as early as 30 weeks. However, if nursing is a struggle, you can pump breast milk almost immediately and preserve the precious colostrum for when your baby is ready. Colostrum is the first stage of breast milk often referred to as "liquid gold." The nutrients and antibodies it supplies are unavailable from any other source. As soon as the baby is stable, all mothers can practice skin-to-skin, which offers intimate bonding time and has been shown to inhance growth and development.

Breastfeeding may not work for everyone but it is worth a try. There are plenty of resources and organizations to help. Many hospitals offer lactation consultants who can help with breast pumping and feeding your newborn right in the NICU. If a lactation consultant is not available in your hospital, contact a local La Leche League leader or chapter. Please visit my website for more resources, information, and links on the benefits of M.O.M. (mother's own milk). You are not alone.

About the Author:

Danielle Leibovici was born and raised in Los Angeles, California. Danielle is a Licensed Marriage Family Therapist, speaker, advocate, former NICU parent, and best-selling author of the multi-award-winning children's picture-book series, **Under The Tree**. Her personal stories and experiences as a psychotherapist and parent, have inspired her books, speaking engagements, and fundraising campaigns.

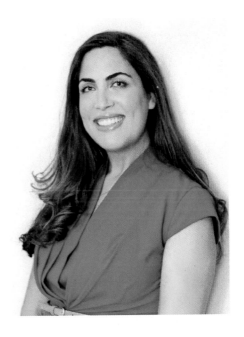

The Under The Tree Series has received the *Seal of Excellence* from the Mom's Choice Awards and her titles include: *If You Love Me So Much, With You Always*, and *Under The Tree.* With beautiful, lifelike illustrations, and supplemental materials, each book connects and inspires readers, young and old, to share their own stories.

Danielle's passion is to help children and adults gain a healthier perspective in life, through honesty, humor, and shared connection. Danielle resides with her husband, three children, and dog in Norfolk, Virginia.

For more information on additional resources, fundraising campaigns, speaking engagements, and author's visits, go to **DanielleLeibovici.com** or e-mail **info@DanielleLeibovici.com**.

Connect with Danielle online. She would love to meet you!

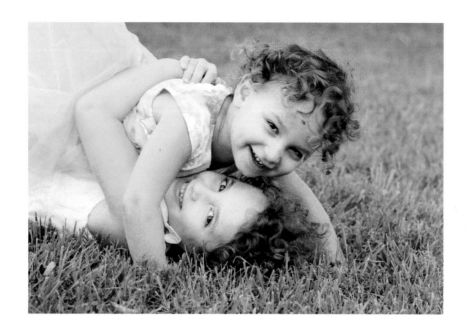

Acknowledgements:

I would like to personally acknowledge and thank the doctors and nurses at Children's Hospital of The King's Daughters in Norfolk, Virginia for the quality of care and compassion they not only gave our own NICU baby, but for the care and compassion they gave us as well. Thank you especially to Ashlynn Baker, BSN, RN, and Allison Ohana, MD, FAAP for taking the time to provide educational information and insight on the greater NICU experience for so many families. I want to thank other NICU mothers and fathers as well, like Darren and Debbie Sigal, for sharing their personal experiences and perspectives on the journey with their children. I would like to acknowledge my husband Sam, my eldest daughter Ava, my mother Jeanne, my close friend Dalia, and my mentor of blessed memory, Nancy Mansfield. During our time in the NICU, we came together and created a safe space that allowed a wide range of emotions and experiences to be processed by all. And finally, I acknowledge and honor Aura, our own warrior baby who taught us to live in the moment, to focus on what we did know, to breathe and to be grateful. You teach us so much every day, and the journey you have made only underscores your resilience and spark for life.